Fightback

FIGHTBACK

MY BATTLE AGAINST MULTIPLE SCLEROSIS

Eli Morowitz

As of press time, the URLs displayed in FIGHTBACK link or refer to existing Web sites on the Internet.

ISBN: 1512115223
ISBN 13: 9781512115222
Library of Congress Control Number: 2015907795
CreateSpace Independent Publishing Platform
North Charleston, South Carolina

For Miliana, Philip, and Rachel—

The core of my universe

Conformity is not necessarily a virtue
Hard work is almost never a vice
Optimism is a moral imperative
And a sense of humor helps.

Harold J. Morowitz

CONTENTS

PROLOGUE

I have PPMS (Primary Progressive Multiple Sclerosis) and I am doing great. MS is classified by medical science as an incurable, progressively degenerative, neurological disease. PPMS is considered by many to be the most severe form of MS. Altogether a fairly gloomy prognosis, if one buys into it.

I was diagnosed with MS over fourteen years ago and at the time of my diagnosis I didn't even know what MS was. Then as I started to learn more about the disease, things got very depressing. The conventional medical wisdom considers my condition to be a one-way trip down the drain. For the first few years after my diagnosis, they had me convinced that this was the case, but then through some good fortune and persistence, I was able to work out a strategy to keep one step ahead of the progression.

When my doctor originally gave me the diagnosis of MS, it was clear that he was really upset about it. I realize now that that was because he knew what the conventional medical wisdom was on MS. I bravely told him to relax, that I could deal with this, because I had no idea what I was getting into.

I was forty-nine years old when diagnosed, and I was going downhill fast. Up to that point I had been a workaholic. Eighteen months after my diagnosis things had gotten to the point where I had to fire myself and shut my business down. I dedicated myself to fighting my MS on a full-time basis.

I started by walking four miles each day and this quickly became six miles per day. Despite all this walking, after just a few short months my condition had deteriorated to the point where I had to start using a cane while walking. Then I had to get a better, stronger, and more stable cane, but I continued hobbling six miles each day.

The only positive at this point was that I was getting the opportunity to get to know my kids better before they left the nest. This disease has also brought my wife and me closer together. Unfortunately, MS drives many couples apart, but my wife has stuck with me through the good and not so good. I don't think I would have been able to successfully deal with my MS on my own.

I was definitely starting to believe that my walking days were nearing an end. My stubbornness combined with my unwillingness to accept the prognosis that the conventional medical wisdom assigned to my condition led me on a journey to find ways of dealing with PPMS, beyond what my doctors were telling me.

I have been blessed with the highest-caliber medical team on my side. But multiple sclerosis is a disease that has not been easy for medical science to figure out. Incredible progress has been made, but it is still largely a mystery.

I will describe how I developed my "kitchen sink" defense, in which I have thrown every available therapy at this disease, and what has worked and what has not. Some alternative therapies, specifically focused exercise including physical therapy, Pilates, yoga, and daily walks, are critical to my defense, and I will detail how the importance of these therapies became obvious to me.

It is my hope that by telling the story of my search, I will be able to assist others in waging an effective battle against this disease.

DIAGNOSIS

Multiple Sclerosis is a wacky disease. For starters, there is no definitive way to diagnose MS, so it has to be done through a process of elimination. This often leads to a long and drawn-out diagnosis process. That was certainly the case with me.

Looking back, it is clear to me that I have had this disease for at least thirty years, but for most of that time I was running through life too fast to notice. Finally, one morning at forty-eight years of age, I woke up with two numb feet. I still tried to ignore it for a few months, figuring that this would clear up. But it did not clear up, and the numbness spread and was accompanied by other seemingly bizarre symptoms. I finally went to see a doctor, who had no immediate diagnosis but ordered several tests, including lumbar magnetic resonance imaging

(MRI). He spotted something on the MRI that he thought might be responsible for my numb feet and referred me to a neurosurgeon.

It took me three months to get an appointment to see the neurosurgeon. He looked at the MRI and told me that what my doctor had spotted was not the problem, and he ordered a thoracic MRI. It took a few months to get the thoracic MRI and get back in to see the neurosurgeon. He told me that the MRI was clean and referred me back to my doctor.

I was a bit frustrated by this point, and I just ignored my numb feet for another couple of months. My symptoms eventually got to the point where I could no longer pretend that everything was fine, and I went back to see my doctor. He examined me and ordered an MRI of my brain.

In the MRI, the gray matter of my brain looked like Swiss cheese. Based on that, he told me that I had MS. As my doctor was giving me my diagnosis, it was clear that he was very upset about it. I bravely told him to relax, that I could deal with this. Of course, at that point, I had no idea what MS really meant. I guess that ignorance can be bliss. (A few months later the doctor confided in me that he had actually suspected MS from the beginning, but that he really wanted it to be something that he could cure. He was a really good doctor and a very nice guy.)

My doctor settled down and continued to deliver his diagnosis and then referred me to a neurologist specializing in MS at a nearby medical school. The first appointment I could get was four months out. Meanwhile, my symptoms progressed. I had developed drop foot on my left side, and bladder control was becoming problematic. Drop foot is the inability to raise the foot sufficiently with each step. In my case it resulted in my left toes frequently catching on the ground as I was lowering my foot, which led to my sometimes tripping on my left toes and the left toe of my shoes wearing out in just a few weeks. After a couple of months of continuing MS problems, my doctor sent me to a local neurologist, whose schedule was much more open.

This neurologist was a bit senile and not up to date on the latest advances in the field of

MS. I had visited him once before when my primary care doctor was trying to diagnose my problems. He had sent me to this neurologist for an electromyogram (EMG) test on my legs. I did not realize it at the time, but the equipment the neurologist used for this test was antique. He inserted huge needles, more than a foot long, into my legs. He didn't stick the needles in far, but once they were in they would hang and flop around. This was already quite uncomfortable, and then he sent electrical impulses into the needles, some very painful. He was looking at a gauge and reading off results to a nurse who was writing them down. At one point he nearly levitated me off the examination table with an extended painful electric shock. Several years later I was administered the same test, but this time by a much younger neurologist using modern equipment. There were no long needles, just small clasps, and just the slightest discomfort, never any pain. The equipment provided a printout of the results. Welcome to the twenty-first century.

I already had reason to be somewhat wary of the local neurologist, and this postdiagnosis appointment ended up being one of the worst medical appointments I have ever had. The neurologist tried to make a game of pulling the MRI sheets out of the folder one at a time and having me guess what I was looking at. He then did some neurological testing, the final step being to ask me to walk for him, in his cramped office with chairs in my way. He laughed at my walking and made light of my other symptoms. He told me that there were some treatments available, but that there were side effects and he really was not too familiar with the drugs. He then went to his bookshelf and pulled out a book on MS and told me to read it. I left knowing that I would never set foot in his office again.

I read the book, which was out of date and scary but affirmed my decision to avoid that neurologist in the future.

When my appointment with the MS specialist at the nearby medical school finally came up, it went much better. This neurologist also did some neurological testing and looked at my brain MRI. He told me that I probably had MS, but that he needed to run some more tests to rule out any other possibilities. In anticipation of the diagnosis of MS being confirmed, however, he gave me an information package for each of the ABC drugs, Avonex, Beta-seron, and Copaxone. He ordered a number of blood tests and told me to review the information on the ABC drugs and come back in two weeks with a choice.

I had my homework, and for two weeks I reviewed the information packages, read the material, and watched the DVDs. All three of the drugs were injectables, which did not thrill me. Avonex and Beta-seron were both interferons, with Avonex being a weekly intramuscular injection and Beta-seron being a subcutaneous injection every other day. What turned me off to these choices was the common and expected side effect of flulike symptoms. Copaxone was a daily subcutaneous injection, but with a significantly lower chance of side effects that would interfere with my life. As for which was most likely to be beneficial, nobody knows in advance, which is why the neurologist left the decision to me.

When I returned, after two weeks, he confirmed my diagnosis of MS. He wrote me prescriptions for Copaxone, as well as amantidine for fatigue and oxybutynin for bladder control. He then sent me on my way and told me to come back in six months.

POSTDIAGNOSIS

When I returned in six months my condition was continuing to slide downhill. The doctor made no changes to my treatments, but he told me that things were happening too fast for us to wait six months for another appointment. He told me that we needed to get together again in three months. He wrote that on my folder, handed it to me, and told me to take it to the front desk and make an appointment on my way out. I did as instructed, and the person manning the front desk started banging away on the computer in front of her. She frowned and said, "I am sorry, but there are no available appointments in three months." I asked her when the first available appointment was, and she once again banged away on the computer. She finally determined that the first available appointment was six months out, and she wrote me up for that appointment.

Upon returning to my office, I immediately e-mailed the doctor and told him what had happened. There was no response. I was self-employed and the three-year lease on my office and warehouse was going to expire before my next appointment. I did not yet have any clear idea of what my prognosis was, but it was getting very difficult for me to hold my company together with my symptoms progressing at a rapid pace. I once again e-mailed the doctor, explaining that it was imperative that I get to see him sooner than my appointment in six months. This time, I received a response. He was sympathetic about my advancing symptoms, but he did not address the appointment problem.

I decided that enough is enough and launched a search for another neurologist. One of the Web sites that I was visiting on a regular basis was that of the local chapter of the National MS Society. While poking around their Web site, I discovered their Professional Advisory Committee. I spotted a familiar name on the roster for this committee; it was the doctor who had delivered our son some 13 years earlier.

I knew this doctor better than one might have expected. My son arrived during the World Series, and our favorite local team was in the series, and we had tickets. In fact, my wife and I watched some of the away games on TV in the hospital while she was enduring 50 hours of labor. Several times nurses came in and turned off the TV, saying, "You don't want to be distracted by that." To which my wife yelled back, "Of course I want to be distracted; turn the game back on."

Anyway, after my son finally arrived, it was clear that my wife was not going to make it to the home game the next night. I asked the doctor if he would like to join me at the game, to which he responded, "Of course." I was too lost in the clouds over the birth of our first child to be really coherent at the game, but the doctor and I watched the Oakland A's go down to an ignominious defeat.

When I found this doctor's name on the roster of the local MS Society's Professional

Advisory Committee, I gave him a call, explained my problem, and asked him if he could recommend a good neurologist. He said, "Absolutely," and gave me the name of a neurologist also on the committee. He said that he would call the neurologist's office to advise them about his referral, and then I should call for an appointment. I called somewhat apprehensively but was pleasantly surprised when I was able to get in just a few weeks later. I hoped that this was going to be different from my experience with the medical school.

My first visit confirmed that life would be different with this neurologist. First, I had to wait well over an hour past my scheduled appointment time to see the doctor. I later discovered that that delay was slightly better than average for this neurologist. When I finally met with the doctor, I was favorably impressed. She spent a good deal of time with me, explained a lot about MS that I did not know previously, and explained all of the available treatment options. She also told me, with a big smile, that I was the first male patient referred to her by an ob/gyn doctor.

She asked if the amantidine I was taking for fatigue was helping. It wasn't, so she wrote me a prescription for Provigil. Provigil took a little getting used to but was quite effective, and I have been on it ever since. She also started me on pulse steroid therapy, in an attempt to slow the progression of my MS. She also told me to see my internal medicine (primary care) doctor and ask about preventive therapy for osteoporosis, which can occur with steroid therapy.

Before my first steroid treatment, my primary care doctor sent me for a bone density test. Based on the results, I was told that I had osteopenia, the precursor to osteoporosis. I later found out that reduced bone density tends to occur with MS. This condition has since gotten worse, and I have been on calcium supplements since that first bone density test. But it is interesting that, despite numerous falls over the years since then, I have never broken a bone, as far as I know.

A couple of months after the first visit with my new neurologist, I fired myself and shut down my business. The fatigue and bladder control issues had been making work quite a challenge. My weakened left leg also made it extremely difficult to depress the clutch pedal on the company truck. Whenever a driver would miss a day, which happened frequently, I would have to cover for them. My lease had run out, and I was not going to make the mistake of renewing for another three years.

Instead, I dedicated myself to fighting my MS on a full-time basis. I started walking six miles a day in the hope that that would enable me to keep walking. I also started doing daily crossword puzzles and playing Scrabble with the family as much as possible to help push back against some of the cognitive decline I was experiencing. About that time, my neurologist sent me for neuropsychological testing. I do not remember the details of the results, but I am sure that they indicated that I was losing it.

After a month of daily six-mile walks, I needed to start using a cane. The more difficult the walking became, the more determined I was to keep doing it.

The pulse steroid treatments were great for about 24 hours, and then I was back to the same condition I was in before the infusion or pills. After six months we gave up on the steroids, and I have not had any since. I was then moved onto Novantrone infusions once every three months. The first couple of times there seemed to be some improvement, but that subsided. Novantrone is an interesting drug in that it can damage the heart if continued for a long time. There is a lifetime limit of about 12 infusions, to protect the heart from damage. My neurologist stopped the Novantrone after four infusions. My heart was tested at the end and fortunately there was no damage, but there was insufficient benefit to take any more risk.

I realized that we were running out of options, and at that point my neurologist suggested that I might want to try the Swank Diet. I had never heard of the Swank Diet before, and she explained that it was a diet developed by the neurologist Roy Swank in Oregon in the 1950s. A patient who had moved from Oregon and had been on the diet for over 30 years and was doing quite well had recently visited her. She told me to visit their Web site for more details.

After looking into it I decided to try the Swank Diet. It certainly wasn't going to do me any harm, and in fact it is an incredibly healthy diet for anyone. I had been warned that it was also an incredibly difficult diet. It took a bit of getting used to, but I have never found it to be that difficult. Swank's primary rule was to limit saturated fats (fats that are solid at room temperature). Saturated fats are to be kept at less than 15 grams/day. Consumption of mono- and poly-unsaturated fats is to be kept between 20 and 50 grams/day, depending on activity level. Because I was walking six miles/day and doing other exercises, I have never worried about the level of unsaturated fats in my diet. My diet has been no red meat, no pork, and no dairy products.

Breakfast is usually a bowl of high-fiber cereal with a banana and soy milk. My favorite lunch is another banana, with almond butter, which has half the saturated fat of peanut butter, and I wash it down with soy milk, followed by an apple. Dinner is generally a salad with some skinless and boneless chicken breast or fish. Edamame (soybeans) is a frequent addition. With dinner I always have at least two tall glasses of water to rehydrate myself, after limiting my fluid intake most of the day to limit bladder problems. Lately, my wife has started cooking some excellent vegetarian dishes. A nice hot dinner is especially appreciated after a cold, wet winter day.

The Swank Diet recommends supplementing one's diet with cod-liver oil on a daily basis. These days, cod-liver oil is available in gel caps, so taking it is not unpleasant, as it was when I was a kid. After more than three years on the Swank diet, my neurologist recommended that I replace the cod-liver oil with omega-3 fish oil. I did so and have continued to do so.

I had been to presentations by medical researchers over the previous two years, and two of them from different medical schools had both talked about the possible beneficial effects of statins. One of them discussed the beneficial combination of Copaxone with statins. I was spending a lot of time on the Internet following current research on MS and had seen a couple of clinical studies that had found a disease-modifying benefit from the use of statins. The researchers presenting the results of their research always ended by saying, "Now don't go and ask your neurologist for statins, because the research is still preliminary." But when one finds oneself losing the ability to do one thing after another, and one therapy after another is of no benefit, one may not have the patience to wait years and years until a line of research is completed. In evaluating possible therapies to battle my MS, the single biggest consideration was how likely was a given therapy to do me harm.

After discovering that Lipitor was the most widely prescribed drug in the country and convincing myself that the risks were minimal, I asked my neurologist what she thought of my trying Lipitor as a disease-modifying drug. She initially was not receptive, but I kept pushing for it, and she finally wrote me a prescription for it. Thus, 80 mg of Lipitor was added to my daily drug regimen, and I have been on it ever since.

By this point, it had become difficult for me to walk anywhere without my trusty cane. I was starting to believe the conventional medical wisdom that I would soon need a wheelchair to get around. I would get up every morning and go out for a four-mile walk on the BayTrail. Late in the afternoon I would go back out for another two miles.

I have heard a number of people say that the San Francisco Bay Area is a great place to have MS, and I wholeheartedly agree. The moderate climate is really helpful. There are very few days during the summer that are un-bearably hot. It is never cold enough to find ice on the ground, which is fortunate when you are already tipsy from balance problems. The BayTrail, which nearly circles the San Francisco Bay, is the perfect place to walk. There are no curbs to climb up and down, and it is paved and level. I am able to walk year-round. With my rain slicker, waterproof pants, and water-proof shoes, I can walk in any weather that may pop up.

One of the really nice features of the BayTrail is the wildlife. Once in a blue moon, a harbor seal cruises around close to the shore, but the shorebirds are the most entertaining. There is everything from ordinary sea gulls, to a wide variety of ducks, to great egrets. I once came within just a few feet of a great egret that was just standing next to the trail. My favorites are the pelicans. They are large and cruise at 50 feet, or more, above the water. When they spot a fish, they dive and hit the water with a big splash. Then they sit there in the water for a few seconds and tip their head back so the fish will slide down their throat.

MY EPIPHANY

One morning, after my walk, I arrived home and found our emptied trash cans on the curb. While moving the trash cans off the sidewalk, I tripped and fell. I tried to stand up but could not! I thought, "Oh, my MS has finally done in my walking." I kept trying to stand up but would immediately collapse as soon as I got on my feet. This was getting awkward. Nobody else was around, and I was sitting on the sidewalk, cursing my fate. I finally managed to get to my feet and throw myself across the top of one of the trash cans. Then using the trash can as a walking aid, I was able to slowly hobble and drag the trash can to my door. Once inside, I got one of my canes and was able to move around, but I was very unsteady on my feet.

Later that day, I went out and ever so slowly hobbled my way for two miles of my afternoon walk. The next morning I was dragging myself along on my four-mile morning walk, when I met a friend. The first thing she said to me was, "You do know, you have a badly sprained ankle?" When I expressed surprise, she told me to look at it. I had not noticed previously, but my left ankle was swollen in a rather impressive fashion. My ankle was numb enough that I had felt no pain from the sprain. Feeling rather foolish, I stumbled through the rest of my walk.

When I got back home, I dug around and found an Ace bandage. Upon wrapping my wounded ankle tightly in the Ace bandage, I was instantly able to walk better than I could before the sprain. Well, this was certainly interesting. I did my afternoon walk and again the next morning with no problem, with my ankle tightly wrapped. I then called and made an appointment to see my primary care physician.

When I met with my doctor, I explained what had happened and then I told him that I needed some exercises to strengthen my ankles. He said, "Great idea, Eli, physical therapy." He wrote me up for four weeks of physical therapy and sent me on my way.

When I first visited the physical therapy clinic, I gave the receptionist my paperwork, which included a list of medications I was taking. When she saw the list, her eyes lit up and she said, "You have MS?" I confirmed that I did indeed have MS, and she smiled and told me that so did she. We traded a few MS stories, and she assured me that the physical therapists there would take good care of me. This was my first hint that I was a member of a community of people banded together by MS.

The physical therapists at that clinic did not have a tremendous amount of experience with MS, but they certainly knew their anatomy and how the body moved. They quickly pinpointed the muscles that had atrophied as a result of my MS gait and set to work directing me on how to strengthen them.

After about two weeks of physical therapy, it was clear that moving around was getting easier. By the end of four weeks, it was obvious that physical therapy had been a great idea. For the first time since my diagnosis, my condition was clearly improving. I went back and saw my doctor, and he was excited by the positive results. He asked me if I wanted more, and I told him, "Absolutely." This led to several months of physical therapy, which resulted in a slow but clear improvement in my mobility, as well as my mental attitude. I was given daily exercise routines by the physical therapists, and I continued with these to keep building my strength.

As recently as twenty years ago, people with MS were told not to exercise because it would aggravate their condition. Although it is true that exercise heats up the body, which slows message transmission in nerves and for most people with MS, this results in a temporary aggravation of symptoms; there is a wealth of evidence that exercise can be extremely beneficial in delaying the long-term progression of disabling symptoms. In addition, I have discovered ways of mitigating increases in body heat due to exercise. After intense exercise a cold shower revives me. On the rare hot days around here a cold shower is always a good way to drop my body's temperature back to where I can function okay. I always do my BayTrail walks in shorts and a tee shirt except when it is raining, in which case I put on my rain slicker and my waterproof pants over my shorts. On cold days I am fine in shorts as long as I add a fleece jacket to keep me warm enough.

About that time, a new sports club opened just a few blocks from my home. I signed the whole family up and started making regular visits. My daughter was in high school and rowing on a crew team. This motivated me to add erging (working out on a rowing machine) to my daily workout. I did a 2K erg every day, and for some time I was able to keep my erg times just ahead of my daughter's. Eventually she snuck past me and then blew way past me. It was disappointing, but I had to realize that I was past my peak and she was far from reaching hers. It was an enjoyable competition, while it lasted.

Then our health club started offering Pilates reformer classes. Pilates was developed eighty or ninety years ago by Joseph Pilates, as a rehabilitative therapy. It focuses on core strength, and, as I soon learned, all motion starts with one's core. Because I was somewhat tipsy from MS-induced balance problems, they made me take some private lessons before letting me into a group class. But, after three private sessions, they decided that I could handle a group class. I have continued to this day with either one or two classes per week, except for a short and traumatic break because one instructor decided that my disability made it too dangerous for me to participate. That resulted in a two-month break, but since then I have been a regular.

After a few months of Pilates, the benefits were quite obvious. While on my long daily walks, my drop foot would start to drag as I got tired. All I had to do was tell myself, "Tighten your core," and my drop foot would come up just like it was supposed to.

I have never been able to understand why so few men take Pilates. I recently picked up a magazine called *Pilates Style*. It is written for Pilates instructors, and that particular issue was focused on how to attract men into your Pilates practice and then how to keep them coming. In the magazine, a male Pilates instructor offered the suggestion that instructors create all-male classes. This I found mind-boggling. What heterosexual male would prefer to take Pilates in an all-male environment as compared with the roomful of delightful women I routinely join for Pilates. My wife frequently joins me for Pilates, and we both think it's great.

A little more than five years after I started my first physical therapy, I was finally able to walk without a cane. I still carry it around in my car as a kind of security blanket, but I have not used it once since that point more than four years ago.

A few years ago, my wife convinced me to try yoga. She has been practicing yoga regularly for more than fifteen years. It helped with both my balance and coordination, and, much to my surprise, it was fun. Since then I have practiced yoga on a regular basis.

I was noticing some cognitive issues, such as turning in the wrong direction while driving just a few blocks from home. My memory was becoming a problem, and I was having frequent "senior moments." After first suggesting that it might just be a function of my age, not my MS, my neurologist prescribed a couple of medications to address the problem. I also got more intense in my work with crossword puzzles and started doing sudoku puzzles. I also visited Internet sites with games designed to exercise one's brain. The combined effect has been a dramatic improvement in my mental acuity. I still have memory lapses and some senior moments, but I am much more clearheaded and navigate in familiar territory without a problem.

VITAMIN D

About three years into my recovery, there was a new MS self-help group starting up nearby, so I decided to go to a meeting to see what it was about. It was pretty much as billed: a group of people dealing with a common malady, getting together to share their experiences. I found it useful and became a regular attendee. A few months after I joined, the group leader hooked up with a local endocrinologist, who was big on the benefits of vitamin D. This doctor had a history of treating diabetes and even some cancers with massive doses of vitamin D. He did not have a lot of experience with MS, but he recommended that our leader start taking 50,000 I.U. of vitamin D_3/day. He did so and began reporting the beneficial effects to our group.

This was very interesting. Conventional medical wisdom dictated that any dose in excess of 2,000 I.U./day could be damaging to one's health. I started doing some research, trying to find evidence of harmful effects of excessive doses of vitamin D. What I found was a growing body of evidence that many of us were probably suffering from too little vitamin D and scant evidence of any harmful effects of too much of the vitamin. I found a single incident of overdose. A dairy somewhere in New England in the 1980s totally lost control of the vitamin D they were adding to their dairy products. Eventually, with many people suffering from massive doses, it was traced back to the dairy. Once the dairy got things under control, everybody seems to have recovered.

Before visiting the endocrinologist, I had asked my internal medicine doctor for his opinion. He was familiar with the endocrinologist, and he told me that he definitely thought outside the box and that he had been quite successful with some patients. He did not see any great danger, so I set up an appointment and went to visit the endocrinologist.

Not surprisingly, he recommended that I start taking 50,000 I.U. of vitamin D_3 every day. After several weeks of this, I started getting feeling back in my feet, which had been numb for the previous seven to eight years. There was still numbness, but I was able to wiggle my toes again, and to push off with my toes while walking. This was exciting stuff, until after two and a half months of the high dose of vitamin D_3 I started feeling severe fatigue. I returned to the endocrinologist whose reaction was somewhat disappointing. He told me that it might be best if I stopped the vitamin D for a while but provided no particular insight as to what was happening. So I went to visit my internal medicine doctor.

He told me to stop the vitamin D and ordered a blood test to determine what my internal vitamin D level was. My level was off the charts, in excess of 300, with normal between 30 and 100. He said that I should be fine in a couple of weeks, and I was. I then went back on 2,000 I.U. per day, or 3,000/day when I don't get any sun. Through it all and to this day, I have retained some feeling in my feet and the added ability to use my toes. My current neurologist likes her MS patients to keep their blood level of vitamin D around 75. I am now taking 10,000 I.U. per day, which keeps my level between 75 and 100.

The self-help group I attended met twice each month at 2:00 p.m. on Tuesday afternoons. In the first six months of these meetings there were a number of people who came to one or two meetings but could not continue because they worked during the day. Several of them asked our group leader if he might move the meetings to the evening, so it would be easier for people who worked to attend. But the leader liked the meeting time as it was and the group got pretty good attendance, so no change was forthcoming.

I started thinking that I might start up an evening group, so that there would be something available for those who worked. I eventually contacted the local chapter of the National MS Society to see what it would take to start a group. I just needed to get some training and find a meeting site. No big deal, so I did just that. My group is now in its eighth year.

CLINICAL STUDIES

For years I have made it a daily habit to check MS news on the Internet. Several years ago I ran into some Phase III clinical study results for an experimental drug called Fampridine-SR. It had been tested on people with MS, and the study had been measuring leg strength and walking speed for those on the drug versus a control group on a placebo. The study results showed a clear benefit of the drug. I printed out a copy of the results to take with me on my next visit with my neurologist.

I asked her, "Are you familiar with Fampridine-SR?" She gave me a strange look and said, "You must mean Fingolimod." I told her that I had heard of Fingolimod, but that I was talking about Fampridine-SR. She again tried to correct me, saying it was Fingolimod. I said no and handed her the printout of the

Fampridine-SR study. She took a quick look at it and moved on to another subject. I figured that we were not going in that direction and forgot about it for six months.

At my next visit, my neurologist asked me if I was still interested in Fampridine-SR. It took me a minute to remember what she was talking about, but I gave her an enthusiastic reply. She told me that her office was going to be involved in the next Phase III clinical study of the drug, and that if I met the criteria I could participate. I just needed a diagnosis of MS, a timed twenty-five-foot walking speed within a specified range, and I had to pass an electroencephalogram (EEG). I don't remember what the time range was, but I was within it. The reason for the EEG was that there was a known side effect of the drug, which was seizures. They wanted the EEG to determine if I was likely to have seizures. The EEG was rather weird. They put some electrodes on my scalp, covered them with a metal cap, and proceeded to fire a series of strobe lights a few inches in front of my eyes. It was not much fun, but I passed.

It then took some time for the clinical study to come together, but a few months later we were rolling. This was a classic Phase III study, placebo-controlled and double blind. This means that a portion of the participants would get the experimental drug and others would get a placebo that looked identical. Neither the participants nor the doctors involved knew who was getting which.

For two weeks I did not notice any change. Two and a half weeks in I started noticing improvements in both leg strength and fatigue. One of the exercises that I had picked up from physical therapy and was doing daily was lying on the floor on my stomach and raising my drop foot until it was directly above my knee. Now, for anyone healthy, this would be trivial, but I struggled to raise this foot twenty times. I had been doing this for more than eighteen months on a daily basis. Two and a half weeks into the clinical study, this started getting easier. It got so easy that my physical therapist had me strap a weight on my ankle while doing the exercise. Within a few months, I was lifting my foot forty times daily, with a five-pound weight strapped to that ankle.

I also started noticing that I had more energy. For years I had been taking 400 mg of Provigil daily to counter my extreme fatigue. After a couple of months on Fampridine-SR, I cut the amount of Provigil in half and still had more energy on a regular basis than before the Fampridine-SR. Another factor, which had prompted me to drop the Provigil dosage, was that the Fampridine-SR was clearly making it more difficult to get a good night's sleep.

This was a twelve-week clinical study. Then there was two weeks off the medication and another EEG. Then the follow-on study, where everyone received the Fampridine-SR for three years or until the FDA approved the drug. Because of sleeping problems, I frequently skipped the evening dose of the drug. Finally I gave up the evening dose for good. For a number of years I have just been taking 10 mg in the morning. I appear to have retained all the benefits of the drug without any of the side effects. At times I have had to be a bit sneaky about my dosage, because it does not fit with the FDA's tyranny of "one dose fits all."

The Fampridine-SR was finally approved for people with all forms of MS in early 2010. An interesting note is that this was more than twenty-six years after the medication was first tested in people with MS. The initial testing was done at a dose of 80 mg/day, which apparently led to serious side effects, namely seizures, which led to much delay. Fampridine-SR is a sustained-release formulation of 4-aminopyridine, commonly referred to as 4-AP. Before FDA approval, I came to know several MSers who had prescriptions from their neurologists for 4-AP filled at compounding pharmacies. One person was getting his compounding pharmacy to make his 4-AP in a sustained-release formulation. Upon approval by the FDA the drug's name was changed to Ampyra, and it has been marketed under that name since then.

I have been in several other clinical studies relating to my MS. A couple of them involved just having blood drawn with no follow-up necessary on my part. Two clinical studies involved weighted vests to help with balance, which has been a problem for me for some time.

The first of these two studies was designed to determine if wearing a weighted vest would help with balance. I had to do a number of timed walks, which included a U-turn. Then I was fitted for a weighted vest by a physical therapist who had developed the therapy. She pushed me in various directions to determine how I would react. From that she was able to determine where the weights should be placed on the vest. Once suited up in the weighted vest, I again did a number of timed walks. It was quite impressive because it both helped me balance and made walking easier.

Then the most beneficial surprise was when the physical therapist told me that she held a weekly group physical therapy session called MS Exercise and invited me to join the group. By this time the benefits of physical therapy were quite obvious to me, so I started going.

In my very first MS Exercise session, the therapist showed us how to stretch our legs and self-massage our feet. For more than a year before this, I had been having problems with spasticity. At the end of each day when I got into bed, my feet and lower legs would lock up in a somewhat painful fashion. I had thought that this was something that I was just going to have to learn to live with. All of a sudden, I had a defense against this uncomfortable problem. Every night before retiring, I started massaging my feet and stretching my legs. Problem solved! I still do this today, and on those occasions when I forget, my feet and legs quickly remind me. The MS Exercise sessions quickly became an important part of my defense against MS.

My spasticity has slowly worsened, and I have increased the frequency of my stretching and massaging to deal with it. I now stop and stretch halfway through my four-mile morning walk. I have also gotten into the habit of stretching before yoga or Pilates, which helps me get through the session with a minimum of trouble. At one point, I pushed my neurologist for a prescription to ease my spasticity. She wrote it for me, but she warned me to be careful because it might cause weakness, fatigue, or other side effects. To be safe, I took my first dose before going to sleep one night. I did not notice any effect from the drug until I got into my car to drive the next morning. It quickly became apparent that I was having a lot a trouble controlling the pressure I applied to the accelerator and brake pedals. I immediately returned home and I have never taken that medicine again.

The most recent clinical study I participated in involved an Alter-G Tread Mill. The "G" is for g-force or gravity. The treadmill is designed so that your weight can be adjusted. There was a special pair of shorts I had to put on for each treadmill walk. The shorts had a zipper around the waist that zipped into a zipper on the treadmill. Air was then blown in to take weight off my feet. I had to go in twice a week for seven weeks. Each visit involved a twenty-minute walk, during which I could adjust the speed and incline or decline of the treadmill.

It took a bit of getting used to. The biggest problem for me was that the apparatus didn't allow me to use my natural arm positions while walking. I either swing my arms by my sides as I walk or, more recently, since I herniated a disk,

I like to walk with my arms behind me with one hand holding the other wrist. I like this position because it helps to ensure a good extension of my lumbar spine while I walk. But alas, the design of the treadmill would allow me to walk only while holding onto the frame in front of me.

They had me walking at 80% of my weight. I started out walking at 1.5 mph with no incline, and by the end I was able to do 3.0 mph with two clicks of incline. I have no idea how much of a slope that was. Although my treadmill walking improved as I got used to the machine, I never noticed any improvement in my walking off the machine. The study site was almost an hour's drive from home and then another hour back. So on days that I played guinea pig, I had to skip my usual four-mile morning walk. I was not impressed. I prefer my walking outdoors on the BayTrail.

VITAMINS AND SUPPLEMENTS

I am on a variety of medicines and supplements for my MS. These drugs and supplements fall into three main categories: First, disease-modifying drugs; second, symptom-management drugs; and third, vitamins and supplements.

The disease-modifying drug I have been on the longest is one of the MS injectables. The other disease-modifying drug is a statin. Statins are FDA approved for controlling cholesterol, and their use for MS is off label.

The most significant symptom-management drug I am on is Provigil, a neurostimulant. The other symptom-management drug is oxybutynin, which I have been using for years for help with bladder control.

The vitamins and supplements include calcium, vitamin D_3, vitamins C and E, omega-3 fish oil, oil of evening primrose, and most recently melatonin.

Over the years since my diagnosis, I have added several vitamins and supplements: some because of information learned at self-help group meetings and others that have come to my attention through a variety of channels.

At one self-help group meeting, one of the members told us that her urologist had recommended 500 mg of vitamin C, twice each day, as an aid to help empty the bladder. I tried it, and it seemed to help a bit. I have stuck with it ever since, because even though I was not absolutely sure it was helping, it certainly wasn't going to do me any harm.

About one year into my follow-on Fampridine-SR study, I was talking with my personal microbiologist, my dad. He was asking me about the various drugs and supplements I was on. When we got to my high dose of statin, he mentioned that statins not only impeded the body's production of cholesterol, but also impeded the body's production of Co Enzyme Q10, which is needed by every cell in the body. This substance is present in the cells' mitochondria, and it is a component of the electron transport chain and participates in cellular respiration. Ninety-five percent of the human body's energy is generated this way. Therefore, those organs with the highest energy requirements, such as the heart, liver, and kidney, have the highest Co Enzyme Q10 concentrations.

He convinced me to try adding Co Enzyme Q10 to my daily supplements. I did a bit of my own research and checked with my doctors and then started taking 100 mg of Co Enzyme Q10 three times/day, after each meal. My research also turned up that our primary external source of Co Enzyme Q10 is red meats. I had not had any red meat since starting the Swank Diet several years earlier. I had both suppressed my body's synthesis of Co Enzyme Q10 and stopped eating our primary external source. Not a good combination.

It helped with my fatigue right away, and then I noticed that I had started sweating again when hot. I had never noticed that I had stopped sweating, until it came back. This helped increase my resistance to melting in heat, which had become quite a problem. This was all quite logical, because sweating is the natural way we deal with heat. The improvement in my fatigue was significant enough that I was able to cut my daily dose of Provigil in half, once again. This time I went down to 100 mg.

On my next visit with my primary care doctor, I asked why he had never recommended that I go on Co Enzyme Q10 when he prescribed the high-dose statin for me. He explained that now he did recommend it, but that when I first started on the statins it was not yet accepted as a need.

One thing I have noticed when evaluating supplements is that many of them are promoted with the tag line, "and it will boost your immune system." I have to admit that that line sounds great. One is likely to think that even if this supplement doesn't do everything they claim, at least it will boost my immune system. The only problem is that with MS we are dealing with an autoimmune disease. That means that your immune system may already be out of control, or perhaps just misguided. In any case your doctor is probably trying to attenuate your immune system to slow its destruction of your myelin. I have gotten to the point where that tag line guarantees that I will not be trying that supplement.

WORST MEDICAL APPOINTMENT

I have already described one of the worst medical appointments I ever experienced, which was with my first neurologist. The absolute worst medical appointment was less than a year later, with a medical-school urologist. My second neurologist, the medical-school neurologist, referred me because of my ongoing bladder-control problems.

I arrived a few minutes early, and about half an hour after my scheduled appointment a nurse invited me in. She took me to an examination room, checked a few things, and then told me to take all my clothes off and wait on the examination table. I was given a paper gown to cover myself. The nurse departed, leaving the door open. Obviously not much concern for patient privacy, I thought to myself. I prepared myself as directed and awaited the doctor. About 10 minutes later, the doctor strolled in with a student, who was one of the most attractive young women I have ever seen. He introduced himself; there was never an introduction to the student. He then proceeded to tear my gown off and give me a brutal examination. Twice during this examination he went out into the hallway and yelled at someone about screwing up his schedule for the day by something they had scheduled for that afternoon. Throughout this the door was never closed, and the student paid attention during the examination and tried to study the ceiling while the doctor was ranting in the hallway.

He finally settled down and told me that I needed to return for further testing. I got dressed and left, knowing that that was my first and last visit to that doctor. This was less than a year after my diagnosis with MS, and I had yet to get past the denial stage in dealing with it. This incredibly degrading visit was the low point of my MS career. For a couple of weeks I figured that there was not much left to live for.

Then I started getting really angry. How did this jerk end up being a doctor? I had never told my wife about this appointment, but she knew that something was wrong. Eventually, she cheered me up with her wit and charm, and I moved on with my life.

I have a friend with MS who has been seeing that urologist for several years and is happy with him. Perhaps I just caught him on a bad day, but good grief, that behavior was unacceptable for anyone, let alone a doctor.

MINOR MEDICAL PROBLEMS

A few years ago, I started noticing a pain in my heels when walking. In a bizarre sense, this was good news. After years of numb and tingling feet, there was no mistaking the sharp pain coming from my feet with each step. Alas, pain is not good news, and it was getting worse. One morning, on one of my morning walks accompanied by one of my trail friends, I mentioned the pain I was feeling. She asked me if it was just plantar fasciitis, and I replied in the affirmative, although I had no idea what plantar fasciitis was. The term sounded familiar, but it meant nothing to me.

As soon as I got home, I got on my computer and started researching plantar fasciitis. I quickly saw that my symptoms were a perfect fit for this malady. Then I continued looking into how I could deal with this problem. There were a few options, but the most attractive for me was some stretches. I was already doing hamstring stretches several times a day to counter spasticity, and one site recommended a slightly modified hamstring stretch. I started adding the modified stretch to my daily routine. The pain started to subside by the second day, and after four days it was gone for good. I kept doing the modified stretch for a few weeks but then dropped it. The plantar fasciitis has not returned, but should it ever return, I am ready to deal with it.

I then admitted to my trail friend that I didn't know what she was talking about when she first mentioned plantar fasciitis, but that her diagnosis was spot on. I explained how I had dealt with it and thanked her profusely.

One morning while eating my breakfast, I noticed a pain in my chest. The pain was mild, but you know how we have all been warned against ignoring chest pains. I finished my breakfast and got ready to go walking but first called my doctor's office to set up an appointment. I was told that my doctor was out of town but they could set me up an appointment with another doctor. When I told them the reason for the appointment, they ran me through a series of questions, such as how severe was the pain and did I have any other symptoms. They finally agreed that I did not need to rush to an emergency room and gave me an appointment for a few hours later.

I went out walking and then went to see the doctor. Throughout the walk, the pain was unchanged. When I got to the doctor's office, I was shown in to a young doctor who was clearly concerned about my chest pains. She examined me and then ordered an electro-cardiogram (EKG). The doctor left and a nurse came in and wired me up for an EKG. Once this was done the doctor came back in and told me that the EKG was normal and now she wanted me to get a chest X-ray. This was across the hall and was completed within about an hour. Then I went back to see the doctor again. She told me that everything looked normal and she didn't think I was in any great danger, but nonetheless she wanted me to have a sono-gram within the next few days, in an attempt to determine what was causing the pain.

I had the sonogram, and the doctor called me and told me that the sonogram was normal and she asked me how I felt. I told her that I felt fine and that the pain had started to subside. She told me to get back in touch with her if it started to get worse. A little more than a week after it started, the pain was gone. I was naturally a bit curious about what had been causing the pain. I knew I had not been imagining it and I had never had any reason to suspect any problem with my heart. With the pain now just a memory, I felt fine and decided to just forget about the whole episode.

Several months later, while eating my breakfast again, the chest pain returned, and it felt exactly the same as it had the first time. Again the pain was mild but exactly where my heart is located. I called my doctor's office and they told me that he would squeeze me in as soon as I got there. My doctor examined me and could not find a reason for the pain. He told me that it was clear from the tests that had been run the last time I had this pain that my heart was quite healthy and could not be the problem. He suggested that it might possibly be acid reflux. He wrote me a prescription for some drug for acid reflux and told me to come back if that did not help. I got the prescription filled and went home.

That evening I discussed my doctor's visit with my wife. My son, who was home, asked me to show him exactly where I felt the pain. I should mention that my son is a superbly trained massage therapist with incredible insight into anatomy and kinesiology. I showed him the spot where the pain started on my chest and where it ended on my back. He felt the spots and told me that I had a large knot in the muscles in each spot. In just a few minutes he had worked the knots out and my pain was gone.

Now this was very interesting. I started thinking about what could have caused my muscles to knot up painfully. All of a sudden, a light went on. Part of my daily physical therapy routine is using free weights. It occurred to me that a few days before each of my incidents of chest pain I had increased the weights that I was using. I suspect that if I did not have MS screwing up message transmission in my axons, it might have been apparent to me that it was a muscle problem. I had a painful spot on my chest and another one on my back, and it felt to me as if the pain was going right through my torso, from front to back. I e-mailed my doctor and explained what the problem had been. It can be great to have a medical professional in the family.

Back when I was using a cane on my daily walks, I would occasionally trip and go down. Generally this was no big deal. One day I tripped and went down particularly hard, slamming into the pavement on the trail. It knocked the breath out of me, and I was sprawled out on the ground. Stunned, uncomfortable, out of breath, and in some pain, I started gathering myself together, and eventually managed to sit up. At that point a bicyclist came by and stopped. He asked me if I was okay. I was having some trouble talking, but I tried to tell him that I was fine. It was obvious from his reaction that I didn't look fine. I figured I had better get to my feet before he made a big deal out of this, so I stood up. Big mistake. I immediately fell over again. He pulled out a phone and was preparing to call 911. I was able to convince him that it was not necessary and I just needed a few minutes to catch my breath. I kept telling him that I was fine and he could go on his way. I knew that whatever I was dealing with, nothing would ruin my day as much as an ambulance ride and a visit to an emergency room. He finally appeared to believe me and departed.

After what must have been at least another 10 to 15 minutes, I was finally able to get on my feet and stay vertical, with the help of my cane. As I surveyed the scene, I noticed that there was a police car sitting about 100 yards away, with an officer taking care of paperwork. I had never seen a police car parked in that area before, and I realized that the bicyclist must have called our local police department and expressed his concern for my condition. I appreciated the fact that the officer was playing it cool, and I realized that I had better make my departure look good or my day would be ruined. Fortunately I was near the end of my walk and my car was close by. I carefully and painfully hobbled to my car and settled into the seat. The hard part was over. I started up my car and headed home. The nearby policeman waved as I went by. I forced a smile and waved back. Disaster averted!

Once I got settled in at home, I took inventory and it was clear that in addition to some minor scrapes and bruises, I had some painful ribs. I set up an appointment with my doctor for the next day. He quickly determined that I had either bruised or cracked some ribs. He wanted me to get an X-ray, but being the minimalist that I am, I asked him if that was really necessary. He thought about it for a moment, and told me that I could skip the X-ray. He said that the therapy would be the same whether they were cracked or bruised. He then listened to my breathing to make sure that my lungs were okay, and he told me how to deal with bruised or cracked ribs.

After a few days, it only hurt when I moved the wrong way, which was almost any way. The most painful thing I could do was to laugh. My family is usually good for some good laughs, but all of a sudden everything they said was uproariously hilarious. It was a rough six weeks until I healed enough so that I could laugh without pain.

MY KNEES

A few years into my MS career, my neurologist recommended that I see an orthopedic surgeon about my walking and specifically about my proclivity to hyperextend my left knee while walking. This was the neurologist whose office was an hour's drive from my home, and she recommended that I see my primary care doctor to get a referral to an orthopedic surgeon. The referral was made and I called the orthopedic surgeon's office for an appointment. They gave me an appointment, but told me that I needed to get my knees X-rayed first. I did so and went to see the orthopedic surgeon carrying my X-rays.

They set me up on an examination table and placed the X-rays on a light board. A few minutes later, the doctor came in and introduced himself. He then sat down to examine the

X-rays. He asked me if I was aware that I had arthritis in both knees. I told him that was news to me and that I never had any pain in my right knee and only occasionally in my left knee. He then proceeded to examine my knees. I was lying on my back and he first played with my left knee. He asked me if I was aware that my left anterior cruciate ligament (ACL) was blown. I certainly was not. He then checked my right knee and told me that my right ACL was blown too. He said that the damage had probably occurred a long time ago and asked if I had any idea what might have caused it.

I quickly came up with the only incident that I could recall that might explain the damage to my ACLs. On my tenth birthday, my parents gave me a speedometer for my bicycle. The very next day I crashed my bicycle into the only car on the street, which was parked, while staring straight down at my speedometer and pumping furiously. My bicycle was destroyed, and I was tangled up in it on the trunk of the car. Then I slid, with the bicycle wrapped around me, back off the trunk to the ground. I couldn't walk for two weeks. My knees turned black and blue and then purple and yellow. Slowly I healed, and I was never aware that any permanent damage had been done.

The doctor told me that they never used to repair ACLs on anyone over 40, but now they were doing it on people much older than that. I was about 55 at the time of this appointment. The doctor told me that because of my MS, he really was not sure if it made sense repairing my ACLs. By this point it was clear to me that my daily walking and exercise were yielding me tremendous benefit, and I could not imagine what would happen to me if I had to stop walking for weeks or months. I asked the doctor what other treatments were used for blown ACLs, other than surgery. His answer was, "Physical therapy." "Great," I said, "would you write me up for some physical therapy?" He told me he would be glad to, and that led to another extended round of physical therapy.

At the end of that appointment, the doctor wanted to see me walk. That sounded good, since the reason I had been sent to him in the first place was because every medical professional I was seeing was concerned over my tendency to hyperextend my left knee while walking. The doctor watched me walk back and forth several times and began shaking his head. He finally said, "I don't see any hyperextension." I asked him if he was sure, and he confirmed his original observation. I didn't know what to say, but this seemed very odd.

To this day, my left knee is one of the largest problems I have with walking. I continue to work on it, with physical therapy and practice. Every medical professional who watches me walk, except for the orthopedic surgeon, warns me about my tendency to hyperextend my left knee. Ever so slowly I continue to improve, but this likely will be a weak spot for a long time.

MEDICAL EQUIPMENT

Since my diagnosis, I have at times used several different types of medical equipment. These devices have been aimed at improving either my mobility or my balance.

Shortly after I began walking six miles each day, it became obvious that I needed some help to continue these walks. Nobody had suggested anything, and I was really not sure what would help. I poked around and decided that perhaps a cane would help. The next time I visited my neurologist (my third), I asked her if she thought a cane would help. She told me yes, and then I asked her what now seems like a stupid question, "Where does one buy a cane?" She did not seem sure but said, "Don't pharmacies carry canes?" I could not remember ever seeing any canes in a pharmacy, but I told her I would look. Her office is in a college town

with a wide variety of shops, and she then suggested that I check out the two African shops
within a few blocks of her office. She told me
that I should be able to find a sharp-looking
cane at one of those.

Before starting the hour drive home, from
her office, I checked out the two African shops.
Indeed, one of them had a selection of hand-
carved African canes. I selected an attractive
one with an elephant carved into the large
handle and bought it. In the shop I had only
taken a few steps with the cane. When I got
home and tried some distance walking, it was
quickly obvious that this cane was not going
to help. It was heavy and way too long for me.
As I later learned, the length of a cane is absolutely critical in determining its usefulness. All
I knew at this point was that this cane was not
going to help.

I went to my local pharmacy and purchased
an inexpensive wooden cane, which fortunately came with a little instruction manual
on how to properly size the cane. Once I cut
the cane down to the proper length for me,
it turned out to be quite beneficial in helping

me walk. I later purchased a virtually indestructible acrylic cane with a handle at a right angle to the shaft. This became my regular walking partner for the next few years. I still have no idea if my neurologist has any idea as to how to select or fit a cane to one's personal needs.

I have managed to gather a collection of ankle foot orthotics (AFOs) over the past decade. The intent of using these devices was to correct my drop foot. My MS has affected me primarily on my left side. When I walk I have trouble lifting my left foot, which can result in me tripping on my left toes. The AFOs are generally made in the shape of an "L," with the upright portion along the lower leg and the lower portion running under the foot. By keeping the ankle rigid, they assure that when the leg is lifted to take a step, the toes are lifted and do not drag.

I found my first AFO on the Internet for $20. As I later found out, this device was a real bargain. It was quite effective at lifting my toes, and the only problem I had with it was that it became uncomfortable when I walked long distances, as I was doing on a regular basis. I stopped using it because of the discomfort. A bit later, one of my doctors referred me to a physiatrist for my walking problems and because of pain that was occurring in my left knee on my long walks.

This was an interesting visit. The doctor examined me and watched me walking. He asked me what my major concern was, and I told him that it was the pain in my knee while on long walks. His first suggestion was to not walk so much, which made me laugh. I explained to him that I enjoyed walking and that my MS made it crucial that I kept walking so I could keep walking. He smiled and then suggested that an AFO might alleviate the knee pain I was experiencing. He then wrote me a prescription for an AFO.

The next day, at MS Exercise, I told the physical therapist about my visit with the physiatrist. She was familiar with my condition and my defense against it. She suggested that I should make sure that I got a Swedish AFO. The Swedish AFOs tended to be lighter than the custom-made ones, which is what local orthotics shops usually supplied. I dug around and found a couple of models of Swedish AFOs that looked much more likely to fit my needs than a custom-made device.

I booked another appointment with my physiatrist and asked him about the Swedish AFOs. He agreed that they might be a better fit for my situation and he wrote me another prescription, specifically for a Swedish AFO. I then headed out to my local orthotics shop. I handed the orthotist my prescription and told him what I wanted. He then proceeded to tell me why I did not want a Swedish AFO, and that I would be much better off with a custom-made device. I noticed that they had a couple of Swedish AFOs sitting around, and I suggested that he try one of those on me. He then told me how difficult it was to get a good fit with a Swedish AFO and made it clear that the only AFO I was going to get from him was a custom-made device. I finally figured that maybe this fellow knows what he is talking about, and I let him talk me into what I did not want. Making the custom-made AFO was quite a production. He had to make a mold of my lower leg, which made me feel as if I were in some grade-school arts and crafts class. Once that was completed, he told me to come back in a week and my AFO would be ready.

I went back a week later and tried out my custom-made AFO. To start, he gave me a sock, which went up to just below my knee. I put the sock on and then he brought out the AFO and put it on. It was hard plastic and entirely encased my leg from my knee to my ankle. It was split in half and had snaps to hold it together on my leg. It extended behind my ankle, and then it had a flat section to go in my shoe, under my foot. It was quite a hideous sight and felt awkward before I even stood up in it. I tried a few steps and he assured me that I would get used to it, once I walked around a bit. I took it off and foolishly paid the co-pay and left. The device cost almost $900, but fortunately my insurance picked up 90% of the cost.

To stay cool, I walk year-round in shorts, except when it is raining hard, in which case I put on my waterproof pants. When I got home, I put on my AFO and went for a walk. I was overheating quickly and only made it a couple of blocks. I dragged myself home and retired my expensive, custom-made AFO. I now had two AFOs. My $20 model was pretty good but uncomfortable on long walks; and my expensive, custom-made model was useless. This should have been a lesson learned about trusting my own intuition with regard to medical devices, but apparently I am not that bright.

A couple of years ago, I was again advised to get an AFO. I thought my walking was coming along fine, but my physical therapist was concerned that I was hyperextending my knee and was convinced that an AFO would help me stop this behavior. This was long after I had stopped using my cane, and I was convinced that I could continue to improve my walking using physical therapy, core strength, and practice, practice, practice. The next time I had an appointment with my doctor, I asked him about an AFO. He did not have strong feelings about it, but he said that if I wanted one he would be glad to write me a prescription for it. I foolishly figured that I would give an AFO one more try.

My physical therapist had recommended that I go to a specific orthotics office to select my AFO. It was part of the same company as the place where I got my custom-made AFO but in a different city. This office had a selection of Swedish AFOs. I picked out a model that looked useful and tried it on in the office. It seemed to help but was not the right size for me. They ordered one in my size and I went back and picked it up a few days later. It had been six or seven years since I had bought my last AFO, and like all medical items, prices had shot up. This AFO was well over $1,000, but once again my insurance picked up 90% of it.

I actually wore this AFO on my daily walks for a couple of weeks. Ultimately, I decided that it was just more trouble than it was worth. I know a couple of MSers who use AFOs on a regular basis and find them to be quite beneficial. I think the reason that they were not a good fit for my situation was because of the amount of walking and exercising that I do. I think that my physical therapists have just never run into a case quite like mine.

Another type of medical equipment that I have used is a weighted vest to help with balance. I have already mentioned the clinical study I participated in that studied the benefits of a weighted vest on balance and mobility. The physical therapist that developed this hypothesis has actually formed a company to make these vests available to all who can benefit from wearing them. She has also gone through the long and involved process of getting the vests approved by Medicare. When that approval was obtained, private insurance companies then started covering these vests.

Although I found that the vest improved my balance and walking speed, I did not see the justification in buying one. That changed when I herniated a disk in my back. My physical therapist recommended a vest to help with my recovery. The vests are available in both soft-back and stiff-back models. The stiff back helps maintain your posture when walking. I got my doctor to write me a prescription for one, and it was helpful with my recovery from the herniated disk. Once my back was back to normal, I was able to remove the plastic, which converted it into a more comfortable soft-back model. I sometimes still wear this for my long walks when it is cool out. When it's hot, I still go with just shorts and a tee shirt. On those occasional days when it is really hot, I carry a spray bottle of water. I spray the water on my legs, arms, and neck to keep cool on hot sunny days.

GREAT MEDICAL PROFESSIONALS

Although I have described some horrific medical appointments I have had, I do not want to leave anyone with the impression that I have a negative view of medical professionals. The vast majority of doctors, nurses, and therapists are highly competent, well trained, and sensitive. But there are a few rotten apples out there, and if you run into one of them you want to walk away quickly.

Through both luck and hard work, I have the greatest team of medical professionals working with me to fight back against my MS. Since my diagnosis, I have had two primary care doctors, both exceptional. The first decided to open a specialty practice a couple of years after my diagnosis. He referred me to the doctor I have been seeing since then. He is so good that my wife and kids also have been seeing him as their primary point of contact with the medical industry. Having doctors that you can easily communicate with and trust is incredibly important to keeping oneself stress free.

I am now with my fifth neurologist since my diagnosis. As I have already described, the first was senile and not well informed about MS. The second was excellent but did not have the time I needed, because of the medical school bureaucracy he was working in. The third was very good, and I was with her for eight years. The only problem was that she was not always ready to accept new research findings that might not be consistent with what she had learned in medical school. She also did not think it appropriate for a patient to give her a book about his condition, a mistake I made twice. Each time, she took the book and then proceeded indirectly to let me know that she did not want her patients acting as informed partners in the relationship with her. This was totally out of step with my evolving vision of my role in managing my disease. It was time to walk away. The fourth was excellent but moved away.

Each neurologist I have seen has been better than the previous one. I have been with my fifth and current neurologist for a couple of years, and she is absolutely fantastic. She is totally comfortable with her patient being an informed partner, and she is up on the latest research and is a great communicator. She is sensitive and perceptive and has a great sense of humor. What more could one want in a neurologist?

I have worked with a number of physical therapists over the years. Most of them have been really good, two have been exceptional, and a couple of them have been mediocre. One of the exceptional therapists ran the weekly MS Exercise class for close to eight years. The typical class had between six and twelve participants, ranging from mildly impaired to wheelchair-bound. This therapist was able to get everybody exercising and pushing his or her limitations while keeping everyone safe and entertained. These classes were not only beneficial, but also entertaining. It was a great group of people, and everyone there saw benefits from the exercise.

The second exceptional therapist I started working with when I herniated a disk a few years ago. She was able to pinpoint exactly what work I needed to improve my situation and got me quickly on my way to recovery. Once she got my herniated disk under control she moved on to neuromuscular re-education. She understands neuroplasticity and just what I needed to continue improving my mobility.

I have been back for more physical therapy with this therapist, and the benefits have been remarkable. On my most recent round, she identified my weak left quad as the biggest cause of my mobility impairment and set to work to fix it. She gave me exercises to strengthen my left quad and began working on remedial walking instruction. As a result, my drop foot has been virtually eliminated. I am doubtful that most doctors would believe that this is possible. This therapist manages the clinic and is obviously a very talented manager. It is clear that everyone working there really knows his or her stuff and enjoys the work. This makes going to the clinic a real joy.

Also a key part of my team, although not strictly speaking a medical professional, is my Pilates instructor. I have been with the same instructor for more than seven years, and she does a great job of pushing us to our limits every session. No two sessions are exactly the same, and each one feels just a bit more difficult than the previous session. She has also been great about keeping me away from dangerous positions. My poor coordination and balance put me at risk in positions that would not be a problem for most people. I have had instructors that were not careful enough in this regard. She has been a central part of the continuing improvement in my mobility.

I recently took a trip to the East Coast to visit family. The trip caused me to miss three of my semiweekly Pilates reformer sessions. The last few days of the trip I was losing control of my body. Balancing was getting much tougher, bladder control was going south, and although I was doing a lot of walking and step climbing, it was getting harder and harder. Two days after I arrived back on the left coast I had a Pilates session with my fantastic instructor and five other young and healthy people. I walked out of there feeling better already. It is clear that to a large extent Pilates is the glue that is holding me together. Core strength is incredibly important for dealing with my MS.

NATIONAL MS SOCIETY

My first contact with the National MS Society (NMSS) was when my wife brought home some NMSS magazines from one of her customers with whom she had shared my condition, long before I was ready to start sharing it with anybody outside my family. These magazines gave me an introduction to some of the good, the bad, and the ugly truths about MS. It also led me to their Web site and from there to the Web site of my local chapter.

After I shut my business down, I started volunteering at the local chapter's office a couple of days a week for a few hours each day. It was pretty dull stuff, mostly stuffing envelopes. Not only did I feel that it was not a good use of my talents, it was actually difficult for me because of what MS had done to my left side, in this case my left hand in particular. When there was someone else at the table with me, it was generally someone who was there to work off a traffic violation.

The whole family volunteered at several of the local chapter's bike ride fund-raisers, known as "Waves to Wine" because they started at the coast and ended in wine country. One year my wife and daughter decided that the theme for our rest stop would be Mardi Gras. In addition to the drinks and snacks, we had appropriate music and handed out bead necklaces. In addition, my wife walked in several of the chapter's three-day (fifty-mile) challenge walks to raise money to fight MS and assist those living with the disease.

My contact with the local chapter faded out for some time, until I decided to start my own self-help group. As I was training to facilitate a self-help group, I realized that the chapter was under new management and that most of the staff had turned over as well. All of the NMSS staff I have met in the past few years are competent and talented. The chapter president is quite personable and runs the chapter like a well-oiled machine.

Early last year, one of the chapter staff did a presentation for my self-help group. After the presentation we had a conversation. In the course of the conversation it came up that I personally knew both my state senator and state assemblymember. My daughter had also interned in both of their local offices the previous summer, when she was home from college. The result of this conversation was that I was recruited to join a few dozen other volunteers and society staff members for their annual trip to the state capital to meet with senators and assemblymembers to discuss pending legislation.

This was a beneficial and rewarding experience. The evening before our visits with legislators we heard a presentation by Peter Lee, executive director of the California Health Exchange. He was working in the Obama administration when the Affordable Care Act was being written and debated. He gave an impressive presentation on just what would be happening as Obamacare was implemented over the next couple of years. He also detailed what was in the works for the California Health

Exchange. It was clear that California was in the lead in setting up its exchange, and this was very encouraging.

The next day we walked the couple of blocks to the state capitol to meet with our legislators. We broke up into two-person teams for the visits. I was teamed with an incredibly nice and sharp fellow who had participated in the previous year's trip to the capital. In legislative offices that he had visited the prior year, he was greeted as a returning hero.

We were promoting two bills. One would cap annual out-of-pocket expenses for people's medical insurance plans, and the second bill would limit the liberties some insurance plans were taking with their customers on pain medications. Incredibly, some plans required a patient to go through as many as five failure cycles on less-expensive pain medications, each lasting up to a few months, before finally paying for the more-expensive pain medication their doctor had originally prescribed. We received positive feedback to our presentation of the two bills, and the first has been passed by both houses and signed by the governor.

The second is still being debated. Lawmaking can be a long and drawn-out process.

In my own assemblymember's office, we had an interesting visit. We stepped and rolled into the office, and it was bursting with activity. As we were being shown to a legislative aide's office, we passed the assemblymember in the hall and he recognized me. He stopped and spoke with us. He apologized for not being able to meet with us himself, but he was on his way to a press conference.

It wasn't until I got home the next day and saw the previous day's newspaper that I realized why his office was in such a bustle of activity. The prior year there had been a leak in one of our utility company's major natural gas supply lines, which had resulted in a fire destroying a couple of dozen houses and killing eight people. After that, it came to be known that the company had been totally irresponsible in maintaining its gas lines for several decades. My assemblymember had been leading the charge, saying that it was the financial responsibility of the company to rectify the situation, and their customers should not be saddled with those expenses. On the morning of our visit, my assemblymember had an op-ed column in the *San Francisco Chronicle* blasting the utility company and detailing his argument. We were right in the middle of this and did not even know it.

This amazing day was made even more complete when, on my way home that evening, I stopped in the town where our daughter is attending university. I took her out to dinner, and I had the most delicious, Swank Diet–compatible, vegetarian portobello burger. Because the restaurant was only half a block away from the hotel where I would be spending the night, I was able to wash my burger down with the restaurant's own microbrew, which was called "rapture." It tasted that good too. Add this together with a rare chance to visit with my entertaining daughter, making this a sweet ending to a long and tough day.

I have since been recruited to join the chapter's Government Relations Committee. This committee helps set the political priorities for the chapter, and its members are an incredibly hardworking group of individuals, united by some connection with MS. A few members of the committee have decades of experience in politics. One of the most experienced is the chapter's director of public policy. He does not have MS himself but has a close family connection to it. The experience of the long-time political activists is invaluable in providing guidance for moving in a direction that will make things happen.

This year there was another trip to the capital for legislative visits. Our day started with presentations from Anthony Wright, the executive director for Health Access California, and Wesley Chesbro, a legislator whose wife has MS. Both presentations were excellent and really cleared up some questions I had on the issues we were going to discuss on our visits. The expansion of Medicaid, under the Affordable Care Act, leaves much of the implementation up to the discretion of the states. The NMSS wants to ensure that the implementation is done in a way that maximizes the benefits to those who need them, while also funding as much of it as possible with the federal dollars allocated for the Medicaid expansion. Our health-care system is complicated, and there are a myriad of issues to be resolved.

It was another long, tough day but successful and rewarding. My involvement as an activist with the Multiple Sclerosis–California Action Network continues to grow. A couple of weeks previously, I had attended a double open house for both my state senator and my state assemblymember. I find it quite satisfying to be in touch with my elected officials. For the past several years I have written my elected officials on a regular basis to make sure that they stay focused on the important stuff. It is never clear that the letter writing has an impact, but with personal contact the impact is very obvious.

Once again, I finished the capitol visit off with a dinner with my daughter. She will be graduating this June, so I will have to come up with another plan for next year's capitol visit. After a long day of legislative visits, there is no way that I have enough energy left for the long drive home.

I have been walking in my chapter's local Walk MS for the past eleven years. These 5K walks are just a bit shorter than my usual four-mile morning walk, and they are fun events. I have also developed a warm friendship with someone I met on a walk seven or eight years ago. For the first six years, the walk was at a site right next to the ocean and frequently fog-bound. That is just my kind of weather, especially for long walks. Due to a massive public construction project, the walk venue has had to be moved for the past two years. The new walk site was much warmer than the old site, and I would melt away during the walks. Naturally, I complained to the Walk MS manager about the situation.

A few months ago, she told me that they had found a third site for the next walk, and she asked me to join the organizing committee for the walk. A few weeks ago, as preparation for the first committee meeting, I walked the new route with my wife, and it is beautiful. The charming walk manager has cleverly put this squeaky wheel in a position where I will be partly responsible if there are problems with this next walk. But it is all to the good. My only problem with the NMSS at the moment is that I wish that I had more time and energy to offer them.

It is clear to me that most of the local chapter's staff are very talented and could be making far more money in private industry or in government. The more time I spend working with the chapter staff, the more impressed I am with the caliber of the team that we MSers have working tirelessly on our behalf. Also very impressive is the caliber of the team of volunteer MS activists that the society's director of public policy has put together. I have learned much from my involvement with this talented and entertaining group.

The story of how the NMSS got started is fascinating. Sylvia Lawry was the founder of the society. In the 1940s, her brother was diagnosed with MS at the age of 21. The doctor had told them that there was nothing that could be done to treat it. A few years after the diagnosis, on May 1, 1945, Sylvia placed the following ad in the New York Times, "Multiple Sclerosis. Will anyone recovered from it please communicate with patient." The ad generated a number of responses, but they were all from people searching for information on the disease.

Sylvia's frustration with the lack of knowledge about MS, even in the medical community, ultimately led her to found the National Multiple Sclerosis Society, with the ultimate goal of finding a cure. It is clear that without Sylvia's pursuit of a cure for her brother, that goal would be decades further away today than we now find ourselves. One of the values that Sylvia instilled into the society was minimizing administrative and fund-raising expenses to ensure that the largest possible portion of the donated money goes either toward research for a cure or for the care and aid of people with MS. This principle is still clearly a strong priority for those managing the society.

In addition to founding the NMSS and leading it for decades, Sylvia also founded the Multiple Sclerosis International Foundation. The foundation supports MS organizations and research around the world. Dozens of countries have national organizations, with information available in a range of languages. The more I learn about Sylvia Lawry, the more impressed I am with the wide-ranging accomplishments of this incredibly dedicated and talented woman.

GREAT MS PRESENTATION (1)

Since my diagnosis, I have been to two to three presentations each year by neurologists studying MS. Some of these have been put on by one of the two major local medical schools. Some have been National MS Society events, such as the annual meeting of my local chapter. Some have been "educational" presentations put on by pharmaceutical companies. I have stopped going to these "educational" events because over the last decade they have become much less educational and more sales oriented.

These presentations have covered a wide range in terms of usefulness and encouragement. Last year, I attended a presentation that stood out from all the rest that I had attended. It was the most focused and encouraging presentation I had ever been to on MS, and the presenter was not even a medical professional. This presentation had three elements that had been lacking in all of the other presentations:

1. A very clear and precise goal
2. A well-laid-out plan to achieve that goal
3. A schedule!

The presenter was Scott Johnson, the CEO of the Myelin Repair Foundation (MRF). Scott is a successful Silicon Valley entrepreneur who was diagnosed with MS in 1976 at the age of 20. Twenty-five years after his diagnosis, in 2001, he was wondering why after years and years of hearing about discovery after discovery and research breakthrough after research breakthrough, there was still so little available in terms of effective therapies for MS. He carefully studied what was happening and came to the conclusion that the new drug development system was broken.

That conclusion led to his founding the MRF in 2004. The goal of the MRF is to develop a therapy to repair myelin in people with myelin damage. Damaged myelin is the one thing in common across all types of MS, so this goal has profound implications for all of us with MS.

This goal will be achieved using a new paradigm for drug development, developed by Scott. This paradigm uses collaborative research between the top research scientists in myelin biology to share their discoveries in real time. Traditionally, a discovery takes years to get published in a scientific journal, and only then can others in the field validate or progress from the discovery. The academic scientists who have bought into this new collaborative paradigm are sharing their research results on a real-time basis. The MRF also gets these researchers together for face-to-face meetings three times a year.

Then there is the "Valley of Death" between discoveries and FDA-approved therapies for treatment. There are several reasons for this Valley of Death. There are more than 800,000 research papers published each year. It is nearly impossible for the pharmaceutical industry to sort through all of these to locate a few promising candidates to pursue for therapies. Scott pointed out that the academic researchers are also speaking a different language than the scientists working for the pharmaceutical industry. The MRF has its own laboratory, called the MRF Translational Medicine Center, staffed with scientists hired from the pharmaceutical industry to bridge this valley.

The MRF also patents discoveries when appropriate. This will enable them to license a fully protected promising therapy to a big pharmaceutical company with enough incentive to spend the hundreds of millions of dollars that it takes to conduct the Phase III clinical studies necessary for FDA approval.

Finally, and perhaps most amazing, Scott has a schedule for achieving his goal. The goal was to have several therapeutic targets in clinical trials by 2014. That goal was beaten by more than a year. The ultimate goal of having an FDA-approved myelin repair therapy available is scheduled for 2019. This sounds ambitious, given the history of new drug development, but I would not bet against Scott meeting this goal. As a man in need of myelin repair, I anxiously await breakthroughs from Scott's Myelin Repair Foundation.

GREAT MS PRESENTATION (2)

There is a self-help group at the University of California at San Francisco (UCSF) that I go to from time to time. Recently there was a meeting of this group that I attended because of the speaker, Dr. Johan Chan. Dr. Chan is an MS research scientist and recently received a prestigious international award for the research he has been doing.

This presentation was also incredibly encouraging. Dr. Chan has developed a means whereby thousands of substances can quickly be evaluated in the laboratory for their potential to promote regeneration of myelin. He has been able to identify a number of drugs, already approved by the FDA for other uses, that exhibit a strong potential to regenerate myelin. He then selected one that showed very positive results for myelin regeneration and has no negative side effects. This drug was further tested on the mouse version of MS with positive results.

UCSF is in the process of putting together a clinical study to test this drug's effectiveness in people with MS: yes, that would be us. Because the drug is already FDA approved, the long, expensive, and laborious three-phase clinical study approval process will not be necessary. If this six-month clinical study shows the beneficial effects the researchers are hoping to see, our neurologists may be writing us off-label prescriptions for this drug in the foreseeable future. I don't want to get anybody too excited, but Dr. Chan's enthusiasm is infectious. It is great to see someone so bright, energetic, and dedicated to his work moving with all possible speed to help us enjoy a better quality of life.

Unlike Scott Johnson, Dr. Chan is not trying to invent a better way to develop drugs, he is just looking for the fastest possible route to helping us MSers out of a tough spot.

CONUNDRUM

A rather bizarre aspect of this wacky disease is the conundrum of looking so good while feeling so bad. This makes it very difficult for those close to you to understand or appreciate what you may be going through. Most of the symptoms are invisible to others, such as fatigue, bladder control, balance problems, cognitive issues, neuropathy, and others. A major frustration is that almost everything is difficult for me to do, which makes the task of rewiring my brain through constant physical and mental exercise particularly daunting.

I have had a total of three MRIs of my brain, including the first one more than twelve years ago, which led to my original diagnosis. As I have mentioned earlier, in that MRI the gray matter of my brain looked like Swiss cheese due to the numerous large MS lesions. My second MRI was about 18 months later, after I switched from my second to my third neurologist. This MRI was indistinguishable from the first; at least that is the way it looked to my untrained eye. My third MRI was more than six years later and was dramatically different from the first two. The size of my lesions had shrunk dramatically. They were now all down to one-quarter to one-third the size they had been before.

This change is something that nobody has been able to explain to me, but you will never find me complaining about it. It will be interesting to see what has happened if I get another MRI, but there is certainly no rush to do that because they are incredibly expensive and they rarely lead to a change in therapy. My MS has been managed primarily by seeing how new therapies affect my symptoms, and that has been working well.

BALANCING ACT

At times it seems as if life with MS is a non-stop balancing act. Most obvious is the struggle to stay on one's feet when one's proprioception has gone south. Every morning I have to relearn how to walk, with the first few steps being the toughest. After a few hundred yards I generally fall into my stride, and then I am good for several miles. It took me several years to learn that I cannot do certain things, such as continuing to walk forward when looking back because someone has called out my name, or I will meet the pavement. My walking continues to slowly improve, and falls are now a rare occurrence.

Dealing with bladder control is another balancing act. During the day I tend to get just a bit dehydrated to avoid too frequent trips to drain my bladder. Then in the evening at home,

I rehydrate. I had a doctor tell me many years ago that this was not a healthy way to deal with the problem, but I have been doing it for more than a decade with no apparent ill effects. I am certainly not recommending this behavior for anyone else, but it has worked for me.

MS-induced chronic constipation is one of the easiest symptoms to control through diet, exercise, and stool softeners. These, however, can be overdone, which can lead to some urgent trips to the toilet. Everything in moderation seems to be the best policy.

I have told you about the neurostimulant medication Provigil, which keeps my mind operating at a reasonable level through the day. This was a difficult medication for me to get used to. Now I am able to handle it without any problems, as long as I don't take it after noon or else sleep that night could be problematic. I was able to reduce my dosage twice as I started first Ampyra and then Co Enzyme Q10. The balance between being alert during the day and being able to sleep at night has required some adjustments to these medications and supplements over the years.

CONCLUSIONS

From my experience, I believe that the two most important things you can do are to get on a healthy diet and get plenty of exercise.

I am not sure that it matters a whole lot exactly what diet you are on. I have been on the Swank Diet for years, and I love it. I have friends who are on the Paleo Diet and are doing well. I also have friends who are on one or the other and have added gluten free to their diet. You need to find the right diet that works for you. Just make sure that it is healthy and that you can stick with it.

There is increasing evidence that exercise is important to everybody's health. Again, you need to find the exercise that works for you and that you can live with as a regular part of your life. Physical therapy is incredibly valuable because it will focus your exercise where you need it most. I love walking because it gets me outside, it gets my heart pumping, and it makes me feel alive and connected with the rest of the world. Pilates is all about core strength, and all motion starts with the core. Yoga has been quite beneficial for my balance and coordination. I have been told that Tai Chi is beneficial for keeping one's body on the right track. Experiment and find what works best for you.

I am not trying to tell anyone the precise path to follow to successfully battle his or her MS. The path that I have followed has been very effective at stopping, and in many respects even reversing, the progression of my disease. The same course may be effective for you, or it might need to be tweaked to personalize it for you and your own personal variety of MS. I do think it is clear that diet and exercise are central components of any successful MS defense, but you need to discover the right diet and exercise routine for you. Then there are the issues of what medicines and/or supplements you want to use.

In the following section, entitled MS Resources, I review some of the finest books

I have read pertaining to MS, as well as some of the better Web sites at which you can find useful information on the disease. There are many more books and Web sites that you may find useful, and new information is becoming available every day. Get out there and explore. Just don't sit back and let this disease roll over you, because if you are too passive it may do just that. Gather as much information as possible and take control of your MS. I think that for anybody diagnosed with a chronic medical condition it is critically important to educate yourself about the condition.

Joining an MS self-help group can be very valuable. It is a chance to talk with people that understand what you are going through, because they are too. Also, in the course of discussing what is working for various group members, I have picked up a number of valuable ideas over the years. The groups can vary substantially, based on the group's leadership and membership. If the first group you visit doesn't feel right, try another one. If you live in an urban area there are likely to be other groups close by. Those in rural areas will likely have more limited options.

Although I have benefited in numerous ways from my time spent at self-help groups, my secret weapon is my family. I could never have launched or maintained my effective battle against my MS without the strong support of my loving wife and our two delightful kids. My wife has also become something of an exercise fanatic, although she prefers aquatic sports. When our daughter was 14, she started rowing on a crew team. My wife then decided that it looked like fun, and she also joined a crew team. Since then, my wife gets up in the wee hours two to three days each week to go row on the bay with her crew team. She does this on a year-round basis. A couple of years ago, she also joined a local Hawaiian outrigger canoe club. So now she also paddles two to three times each week. Seeing my healthy wife exercising constantly has certainly made it easier for me to sustain the level of exercise needed to maintain my mobility.

It is critically important to equip yourself with a strong medical team. Many people are reluctant to actively shop for good doctors, but it may be the most important service you ever purchase, so do it thoughtfully and carefully. Even if you are being treated by a top-notch medical team, you must take responsibility for monitoring your own condition. Even the best doctor will not have the time to dedicate to your condition that you will. Doctors are human and occasionally make mistakes.

Don't believe all the negative stuff your doctor tells you. Do your own research and confirm information independently. Virtually everything is available to you on the Internet; use it. When using the Internet, be cautious about the source of any information you are looking at. There is a lot of anecdotal information, and there is also a lot of information from people who are trying to sell you something. Learn how to verify the veracity of any information you are reading. I would also be cautious about getting into forums because there are a lot of whiners out there. They are not going to do you any good, nor are they going to help themselves.

Ask your doctor to send you to physical therapy as soon as you notice any changes in your gait or any other physical manifestations of your MS. If the answer is no, demand it. If they still refuse, fire them and go hire a doctor who is looking out for your best interests.

My mantra for years now has been, "Objects in motion tend to stay in motion." I love to walk and I have to keep walking so I can keep walking. To a large extent, this is a "use it or lose it" disease.

Have fun and always remember that laughter is the best medicine. Even just forcing yourself to smile will make you feel better. Try it.

APPENDIX: MS RESOURCES

Books

There are hundreds of books on MS out there. Here are a few that I consider to be among the best.

Exercises for Multiple Sclerosis by Brad Hammler, 2006, Hatherleigh Press

I have been battling multiple sclerosis for years and I have read almost every book I have run into on the subject. This book is by far the best for people who are unwilling to surrender to this disease. Brad Hammler clearly understands that it is possible to delay the immobility and other physical problems that MS can cause by maintaining a focused exercise routine. I had come to the same conclusion myself, and I was delighted to read the experiences of a medical service professional, with extensive experience with MS patients, confirming my strategy in battling this disease. I highly recommend this book to anyone with MS. A focused exercise routine has been the most clearly effective therapy of all the therapies I have tried. If you have MS, this book will show you how to fight back and keep active and mobile. Eventually, medical science will develop therapies not requiring this much effort, but until then Brad has the best strategy to battle MS. Continue with whatever drug therapy you may be on, but add Brad's exercise routine to it.

The Brain That Changes Itself by Norman Doidge, M.D., 2007, Penguin Books

This is the book that introduced me to neuroplasticity and explained to me why my relentless repetition of focused exercises was improving my ability to walk, balance, lift things, and basically help restore some of the function that I had lost as a result of demyelinated axons in my central nervous system. I learned that I was "rewiring" my brain, to incredible beneficial effect.

When the Body Says No by Tracy A. Todd, 2011, Outskirts Press

This book is a must read. The author artfully, humorously, and insightfully describes her journey through life with a chronic medical condition. She entertains with her vivacious wit, while relating how she has lived with neurological conditions since her early teens. The author faces her medical challenges with a positive and inspirational attitude. Indeed, everyone faces unique challenges, and one burdened with a chronic medical condition does not necessarily have it worse than someone else. Nobody would choose to live with a chronic medical condition, but if that is what life has dealt you, make the most of it. The book also describes how a loving and caring spouse, with a good sense of humor, can help to make the journey quite enjoyable. The author also describes the extra stresses that her condition placed on her marriage but how working through those stresses with a loving partner has made their marriage stronger. This book is a thoroughly enjoyable, inspirational, and incredibly revealing story.

Life on Cripple Creek by Dean Kramer, 2003, Demos Medical Publishing

This is a book written by someone who has been living with MS for a long time and has survived in part because of her incredible sense of humor, including a willingness to laugh at herself. That is something we could all benefit from. Dean has been writing about her MS for decades, including a monthly column for MS World. She has recently stopped writing so she can better enjoy her active life. I say to Dean, thank you very much for your writing, and music, and especially for your sense of humor; now enjoy whatever else entertains you.

Complementary and Alternative Medicine and Multiple Sclerosis by Allen Bowling, M.D., Ph.D., 2007, Demos Medical Publishing

Because there is not yet a cure for multiple sclerosis, many people with it eventually search for therapies outside conventional medicine. This can be very beneficial, as I have found. But one should be careful not to push aside those treatments that conventional medicine has to offer, and when considering alternative therapies, one needs to be careful to assess their potential harm. This book presents a comprehensive discussion of just about every alternative therapy out there, along with a discussion of each therapy's potential risks and benefits.

Dietary Supplements and Multiple Sclerosis by Allen Bowling, M.D., Ph.D., 2004, Demos Medical Publishing

If you are considering dietary supplements, something that a majority of the people with MS do, this is the best source I have found for evaluating your various options.

The Empowered Patient by Elizabeth Cohen, 2010, Ballantine Books

This is an excellent guide to how to protect yourself when dealing with the medical industry. As the author points out, most doctors are good, but they are human and occasionally they make mistakes. She also describes just how dangerous hospitals are. This is because there are a lot of sick people there, which can lead to the spread of germs and diseases. Hospitals are also large bureaucracies, which can lead to a myriad of problems. She tells you how to act as your own best advocate. This is an entertaining read. It is a must read for anyone who might someday become ill. This means you.

Courage by Richard Trubo, 2001, Ivan R. Dee

This is a biography of Sylvia Lawry, the founder of the National Multiple Sclerosis Society. It details her founding and leadership of the NMSS, including how she instilled it with a core value of maximizing the benefit of every donated dollar. She is the one person most responsible for putting MS in the crosshairs of the medical industry. This incredibly motivated and creative woman is a real inspiration.

The Multiple Sclerosis Diet Book by Roy Laver Swank, M.D., Ph.D., and Barbara Brewer Dugan, 1987, Doubleday

This details the low-fat MS diet developed by neurologist Dr. Roy Swank. In it, he gives his theories that led him to prescribe the diet for his patients with MS and also presents some clinical evidence of its effectiveness. The information is well presented but will not convince many neurologists because of the lack of a double-blind placebo-controlled study. This is known as the "gold standard" for testing medical therapies. The book also contains hundreds of recipes for following the diet.

Overcoming Multiple Sclerosis by Professor George Jelinik, 2010, Allen and Unwin

This book has a tremendous amount of useful information once you get past the first few chapters. The author has MS, and the book is primarily about the research he has done on MS and how he has effectively dealt with his MS. It takes him quite some time to get to the point, with discussions about his mother's MS and a "spirit" that I just did not get. Once you get to chapter 4 in the book, the author covers solid scientific studies and just about everything about MS. He reviews all of the various MS symptoms and all of the therapies for dealing with MS. His recommendations focus on customizing one's diet and exercising, but he is also open to all of the conventional therapies. The combination of conventional therapies with diet and focused exercise is exactly the tack that I have chosen in fighting back against my MS. The one subject where he seems to have a blind spot is in dealing with fatigue. He says that there are no drugs that are effective in dealing with MS fatigue. I am in contact with a number of people with MS, and many of them are using the generic modafinil, or Provigil or Nuvigil, as I have and have found them to be very beneficial for dealing with MS-related fatigue. I recommend this book as an excellent resource for information on MS. The author has an unfortunate tendency toward verbosity, so you may not want to read it cover to cover.

Web Sites

Again, there are hundreds of Web sites with information on MS. Here are a few that I consider to be among the best. There are many excellent sites not included here. Get out there and explore.

www.nationalmssociety.org

National Multiple Sclerosis Society. This is probably the best starting place for anyone newly diagnosed or anyone just looking for information on MS. Founded by Sylvia Lawry in the late 1940s, the National MS Society has been the largest nongovernment source of funds for MS research in the world. The Web site has excellent information for the newly diagnosed about living with MS and about treatments and research. They also have many programs to assist those of us with MS. You can also locate a local chapter of the society throughout the United States.

www.msif.org

This is the Web site of the MS International Federation, with national chapters in many countries. For those of you outside the United States, this Web site offers you a choice of 15 different languages. It will help you to locate MS organizations throughout the world.

www.ActiveMSers.org

A not-for-profit Web site designed to help, mo-tivate, and inspire those with multiple sclerosis to stay as active as possible, physically, intel-lectually, and socially, regardless of physical limitations. This Web site was created by Dave Bexfield after his diagnosis with MS in 2006. It is informative and stays up with the latest news on MS. Dave documents his incredible personal story, and he has a great sense of hu-mor. This site is excellent for both information and entertainment. It also has links to several excellent videos documenting Dave's story and treatment and struggles with his insurance company.

www.patientslikeme.com

This is a networking site for people with chronic illnesses. It has over 30,000 members with MS. I find this site to be a great resource for information on symptoms and treatments. As with almost all sites I visit, I tend to stay away from the forums because you frequently will run into whiners. Fighting this disease is difficult enough without being dragged down by that sort of thing.

www.mscenter.org

Rocky Mountain MS Center. This is a great site for information on MS, and they send out periodic newsletters, either online or via snail mail, if you are interested. There are some very prominent neurologists at this center, including Allen Bowling, author of some good books on MS.

www.narcoms.org

NARCOMS (North American Research Committee on MS). With over 35,000 MS participants enrolled, the North American Research Committee on MS maintains the world's largest self-reported registry of individuals with MS. Participation in the registry is free, voluntary, and confidential. Information is released to MS researchers in summary form only; participant identity will never be released. They distribute a quarterly publication to participants.

www.medlineplus.gov

MedlinePlus is a gold mine of good health information from the world's largest medical library, the National Library of Medicine. MedlinePlus has extensive information from the National Institutes of Health and other trusted sources on over 900 diseases and conditions. There are directories, a medical encyclopedia, and a medical dictionary; easy-to-understand tutorials on common conditions, tests, and treatments; health information in Spanish; extensive information on prescription and nonprescription drugs; health information from the media; and links to thousands of clinical trials. MedlinePlus is updated daily.

www.msconnection.org

I have warned about forums because they can get depressing. But if you are looking to communicate with others who have MS, this Web site seems to have attracted a very positive community of MSers.

GLOSSARY

amantadine. An antiviral medication that is also used to treat some neurological conditions.

4-aminopyradine. A potassium channel blocker that can improve nerve transmission in demyelinated nerves. Also known as 4-AP.

Ampyra. A sustained-release formulation of 4-aminopyradine that has been approved by the FDA for improving walking in people with MS.

atorvastatin. Generic for Lipitor.

Avonex. Interferon beta-1a is used as a disease-modifying medication to decrease flare-ups and slow the development of disability in people with MS. It is administered via weekly intramuscular injections.

Beta-seron. Interferon beta-1b is used as a disease-modifying medication to decrease flare-ups and slow the development of disability in people with MS. It is administered via subcutaneous injections, every other day.

Co Enzyme Q10. A vitaminlike substance that is synthesized by the body; the primary external source is red meats. Co Enzyme Q10 may help increase energy because it has a role in producing ATP, a molecule in body cells that functions like a rechargeable battery in the transfer of energy.

Copaxone. Glatiramer acetate is used as a disease-modifying medication to decrease flare-ups and slow the development of disability in people with MS. It is administered through daily subcutaneous injections.

Ditropan. It is prescribed for overactive bladder. It works by relaxing the bladder muscles. The generic drug is called oxybutynin.

EEG. Electroencephalogram, a test that measures electrical activity in the brain.

EKG. Electrocardiography (ECG or EKG from Greek: *kardia*, meaning heart) is a transthoracic (across the thorax or chest) interpretation of the electrical activity of the heart over a period of time, as detected by electrodes attached to the surface of the skin and recorded by a device external to the body. The recording produced by this noninvasive procedure is termed an electrocardiogram (also ECG or EKG). An EKG is used to measure the rate and regularity of heartbeats, as well as the size and position of the chambers, the presence of any damage to the heart, and the effects of drugs or devices used to regulate the heart, such as a pacemaker.

EMG. Electromyography measures the response of muscles and nerves to electrical activity. It is used to help determine muscle conditions that might be causing muscle weakness, including muscular dystrophy and nerve disorders.

Fampridine-SR. This was the name used for Ampyra during the Phase III clinical studies for FDA approval. Once approved, the name was changed to Ampyra.

Fingolimod. This was the name used for Gilenia during the Phase III clinical studies for FDA approval. Once approved, the name was changed to Gilenia.

generic drugs. Each drug approved by the FDA has two names: a name assigned by the pharmaceutical company that received the approval and patent protection; and a generic name, which will be used by any other companies manufacturing the drug after the patent protection expires.

intramuscular. A deep injection, directly into muscle tissue.

kinesiology. Kinesiology, also known as human kinetics, is the scientific study of human movement. Kinesiology addresses physiological, mechanical, and psychological mechanisms.

Lipitor. In a class of medications called statins. They work by slowing the production of cholesterol in the body to decrease the amount of cholesterol that may build up on the walls of arteries and block blood flow. It is the most widely prescribed drug in the country. Last year it went generic.

lumbar. The lower back; a lumbar MRI is of the lower spine.

melatonin. A hormone found naturally in the body. It can also be made synthetically in a laboratory. It is used to help adjust the body's internal clock and as an aid to falling asleep.

mitoxantrone. Generic name for Novantrone.

modafinil. Generic name for Provigil.

MRI. Magnetic Resonance Imaging uses electromagnets and radio waves to create images of structures inside the body. Getting an MRI can be a long and loud process, but it is painless and harmless.

myelin. An insulating layer around nerves that acts like insulation around electrical wires. If the myelin is damaged it can slow down the impulses moving through the nerves. It consists of protein and fatty substances.

neuroplasticity. Neuroplasticity occurs on a variety of levels, ranging from cellular changes (due to learning) to large-scale changes involving cortical remapping in response to injury or disease. Through most of the 20th century there was a scientific consensus that brain structure was relatively immutable after a critical period during early childhood. This belief has been challenged by findings revealing that many aspects of the brain remain plastic even into adulthood.

Novantrone. This is both a chemotherapy drug used for non-Hodgkin's lymphoma and a disease-modifying medication in MS. It is infused through an IV.

Nuvigil. An FDA-approved neurostimulant for treating narcolepsy. It is also commonly used to treat fatigue associated with MS.

off-label. The prescription of a drug for a condition other than that for which it has been officially FDA approved.

oil of evening primrose. The oil from the seed of the evening primrose plant. It is a source of essential fatty acids.

orthotics. The use of braces and splints to bio-mechanically assist in supporting and stabilizing parts of the body affected by paralyzed and/or weak muscles.

osteopenia. Low bone mass, not low enough to be called osteoporosis.

osteoporosis. A disease in which the bones become fragile and more likely to fracture. The bone loses density, a measure of the amount of calcium and minerals in the bone.

oxybutynin. Prescribed for overactive bladder. It works by relaxing the bladder muscles. It is generic for Ditropan.

Phase III clinical study. This describes the type of study needed to get a new drug approved by the FDA. These are double-blind, placebo-controlled studies. There may be anywhere from a few hundred study participants to more than one thousand. Some of the participants will be given the new drug, and some will be given a placebo. Neither the participants nor their doctors know who is getting which treatment. It is also referred to as the "gold standard" for proving the efficacy of new therapies.

physiatrist. Physiatrists, or rehabilitation physicians, are nerve, muscle, and bone experts who treat injuries or illnesses that affect how you move.

PPMS. Primary Progressive Multiple Sclerosis. One of the subsets of MS, which are defined by the way the symptoms of the disease present.

proprioception. The body's ability to determine its position and the position of its extremities, without looking.

Provigil. An FDA-approved neurostimulant for treating narcolepsy. It is also commonly used to treat fatigue associated with MS.

spasticity. Spasticity is a condition in which there is an abnormal increase in muscle tone or stiffness of muscle, which might interfere with movement and speech or is associated with discomfort or pain. The degree of spasticity varies from mild muscle stiffness to severe, painful, and uncontrollable muscle spasms.

statins. A class of drugs used to lower cholesterol.

subcutaneous. The term cutaneous refers to the skin. Subcutaneous means beneath, or under, all the layers of the skin. A subcutaneous injection is a shallow injection, just below the skin.

thoracic. Relating to the part of the body between the neck and the abdomen; a thoracic MRI is of the upper spine.